COUCH TO CORE

All YOU NEED TO KNOW ABOUT CORE EXERCISES TO LOSE WEIGHT, TIGHTEN ABS, RELIEVE BACK PAIN AND REBUTTING THE MYTHS ABOUT CORE EXERCISES

By

Neva R. Williams

TABLE OF CONTENT

INTRODUCTION

WHAT IS CORE

The axial (central) portion of an organism's body is known as the core or trunk. The phrase is often understood to refer to the torso in everyday speech, although in academic contexts it also refers to the head and neck. This region of the body is crucial for functional movements, and underdeveloped core muscles might increase your risk of injury.

The main muscles of the core are located in the mid- and lower back, not the shoulders, whereas the hips, shoulders, and neck are located peripherally.

The term "core" is used to refer to a number of muscular groups, not just one.

CHAPTER ONE

WHERE DO CORE MUSCLES EXIST?

The following are the core's primary elements:

Your front rectus abdominis, or "six-pack abs,"the side obliques, internal and exterior

The deepest abdominal muscle that runs across your core horizontally is the transversus ababdominis.

The muscles adjacent to your spine that resemble ropes, the erector spinae

A deep muscle that goes down your spine called the multifidus

The quadratus lumborum, a deep muscle above the hips in the lower back.

The diaphragm, which forms the top or roof of your abdomen and is a breathing muscle.

The pelvic floor muscles, which serve as the base or foundation of your core.

These muscles cooperate to strengthen and support your abdomen.

A more thorough discussion of the core muscles is

Your core is more than simply your abdominal muscles, despite what many people think. In actuality, it's a complicated network of muscles on your anterior and posterior kinetic chains that cooperate to keep you stable, upright, and injury-free while you carry out both routine tasks and exercises.

To keep your spine stable and avoid damage, they say, all of the muscles in your core cooperate with one another. Nevertheless, each core muscle has a specific purpose.

A concise analysis of core muscles are:

ABDOMINAL MUSCLES

The rectus abdominis muscles are two long, straight muscles that span the front of your pelvis to the centre of your abdomen. The trunk flexion, or capacity to bend forward or "curl up," is caused by this core muscle.

During lateral trunk flexion, or bending to the side, one side of the rectus abdominis also collaborates with the obliques and the erector spinae.

OBLIQUES BOTH INTERNAL AND EXTERNAL

One of your side's most extreme abdominal muscles, the external oblique muscles extend diagonally from the bottom portion of your ribs to your pelvis.

The internal obliques, on the other hand, extend diagonally from the pelvis up to the lower ribs, sitting below the external obliques. Both of these muscles are involved in lateral trunk flexion as well as trunk rotation (i.e., twisting to the left and right).

ABDOMINAL TRANSVERSE

The deepest abdominal muscle, known as the transverse abdominis, supports the spine by wrapping around the whole waist like a corset. This core muscle is in charge of compressing the abdomen, such as when you drag your belly button towards your spine.

In order to preserve your spine, it also aids in generating intra-abdominal pressure and deep core stability, which stop hyperextension and overflexion.

INHIBITORY SPINAE

A collection of muscles known as the erector spinae runs vertically along both sides of the spine. These abdominal muscles, also known as the back extensors, let you to lengthen your trunk by rolling up from a forward fold or bending backward into a bridge.

To enable lateral trunk flexion, one side of the erector spinae cooperates with the rectus abdominis and obliques. The right side of your erector spinae would aid in the action if you were to bend to the right, for instance.

GENITAL FLOOR

The coccygeus, iliococcygeus, puborectalis, and pubococcygeus are a set of four muscles that lie at the base of the torso and create a hammock over the pelvic opening to support the bladder, colon, uterus, and vagina.

The pelvic floor contributes to the stability of your spine inside the core.

DIAPHRAGM

Diaphragm is a core muscle.

At the base of the lungs, the diaphragm is a substantial muscle with a dome-like form that contracts and expands during breathing. According to Miranda, this core muscle is crucial for producing intra-abdominal pressure, which is the stiffness required to produce motion and avoid excessive motion in the spine.

Research demonstrates that as you inhale, the diaphragm contracts, increasing intra-abdominal pressure and concurrently contracting the transverse abdominis and pelvic floor muscles.

CHAPTER TWO

FUNCTIONS/PURPOSES OF THE CORE MUSCLES

Essentially, what keeps you upright is your core.

Your spine and trunk are stabilised, and your spine is free to flex and move. Balance and postural support are improved, falls and injuries are reduced, and sport-specific motions that create torque and force are produced.

Stabilisers and movers are the two groups of core muscles that make up your body.

The transversus abdominis, multifidi, pelvic floor muscles, and maybe the diaphragm are members of the stabilising group that work to keep you strong and stable by maintaining intra-abdominal pressure. Your body is not moved or bent by them.

The obliques, quadratus lumborum, rectus abdominus, and erector spinae are the "movers." They assist you in standing up, bending forward, twisting, bending to the side, and more.

To be at your most functional, you need to have the right amount of stability and movement. I often see increased lower back and spine discomfort, as well as damage, in persons who have weak core muscles or "non-functioning" core muscles.

As a result, your spine and internal organs are protected from external pressures like gravity and strong ground reaction forces by your core muscles, which also help your body move.

The core generates internal pressure to remove contents (vomit, faeces, carbon-laden air, etc.) and is utilised to stabilise the thorax and pelvis during dynamic movement.

CONTINENCE

The capacity to hold back bowel motions is known as continence, and weak core muscles may lead to urine stress incontinence, which is the inability to regulate the bladder owing to pelvic floor dysfunction.

PREGNANCY

During labour and delivery, core muscles, in particular the transversus abdominis, are engaged. The Valsalva manoeuvre, in which the thorax contracts while the breath is held to aid, often unintentionally, in movements including lifting, pushing, excretion, and childbirth, also uses core muscles.

POSTURE

Most full-body functional movement, including most sports, is typically thought to have its origins in the core. Additionally, a person's posture is mostly determined by their core. The human structure is designed to absorb force applied to the bones and to channel autonomic force via a variety of joints in the appropriate direction.

A person's spine, ribs, and pelvis are aligned by the core muscles to withstand a certain stress, whether static or dynamic.

STATIC CENTRAL PROCESS

The power of one's core to align the skeleton and resist a force that is greater than the apparent effort is known as static core functioning.

Shooting a gun while lying down is an example of a static core function. The shooter must be able to sink both their own weight and the weight of the rifle into the ground in order to maintain accuracy.

Any effort by the shooter to make the sights move dynamically (by forcing them onto the target rather than letting them aim naturally) may result in a jerky posture in which the sights do not sit stationary on the target.

The skeleton must be in proper alignment to place the rifle (and thus, the sights) on the target in order for the shooter to retain accuracy. Muscles cannot be used to put force on the weapon. Despite being on the ground and quite distant from the rifle, the core is still aligning the spine and pelvis, which are related to the shoulder, arms, and neck.

The spine, pelvis, and rib cage must be positioned in such a way as to prevent unnecessary movement of these peripheral parts. In order for the upper body to be in a position where the upper body can offer a firm, strong basis for the rifle to stay stationary, the core muscles maintain the axial skeleton (head, spine, and tailbone).

A DYNAMIC CORE COMPETENCY

Since dynamic movement must account for both the force of external resistance and our skeletal structure (as a lever), it necessitates a significantly different combination of muscles and joints than a static posture.

Dynamic movement needs more on the core musculature than static movement, which only rely on skeletal stiffness, because of its functional design. This is so that, instead of a static, continuous resistance, the movement may withstand a force that modifies its plane of motion.

Movement results in different functions for muscles, ligaments, innervation, and tendon because the body's bones must absorb resistance in a fluid manner. Among these responsibilities is the capacity to modify one's posture in reaction to changes in motion, speed, and power (the cumulative amount of force resisted).

One example of this is climbing a hill. In order to move in a certain direction and stay balanced on a rough surface, the body must fight gravity. The body is forced to align the bones in a way that balances the body in order to obtain momentum by pushing against the ground in the opposite direction of the planned movement.

Even while it would first seem that the legs are the primary source of this movement, without balance, the legs will only cause the person to topple over. Thus, the primary motivation for walking is to achieve core stability. The legs then move the steady core by contracting their leg muscles.

CHAPTER THREE

TYPES OF CORE EXERCISES

Workouts targeting the core are essential because, while you may only think about your "core" when doing specific ab exercises, you are really using these muscles all the time. When you walk, reach, balance, get out of a chair, or even simply stand up straight, your middle muscles are used. This keeps you stable and supported for almost all of your motions.

If you support your core muscles while lifting to increase your stability and stop you from twisting or arching, any activity may become an abs exercise. Furthermore, a number of exercises that you may not think of as "core exercises" can really work those muscles, especially when you're doing tasks like balancing on one leg, lifting weights above your head (like overhead presses), or in front of you (like goblet squats).

Types of core exercises

1. ONE FOREARM PUSH-UP

You can do a forearm plank anywhere! It's an all-over isometric exercise that focuses on your back, legs, shoulders, and spine in particular. You have to hold a certain posture for a specific period of time while doing isometric workouts. The plank is challenging at any level of fitness since it requires continual resistance to gravity in order to stay upright and maintain your core and body's stability.

How to carry out:

• Rest your forearms on the ground with your elbows just below your shoulders, and extend your hands forward so that your arms are parallel.

• Stretch your legs out behind you while placing your toes on the ground.

• Your body should be in a single, straight line from your shoulders to your heels.

• Contract your whole core, glutes, and quads, and tuck your butt in just a little bit to keep your lower back straight.

• Verify that you are not sinking your hips or lifting your butt up towards the ceiling.

• Maintain a neutral neck position while keeping your gaze concentrated on your hands.

• Hold this position.

2. TWIST IN RUSSIAN.

The Russian twist is a great way to warm up your spine and engage your obliques.

How to carry out:

• Assume a sitting position with your knees bent out in front of you, heels on the floor, and feet flexed.

• With your hands pressed to your chest, bend your back until you feel your abdominal muscles tense.

• Slowly turn your torso from the right to the left.

• Keep your core tight the whole time, and remember to breathe.

3. SIT-UP BUTTERFLY

When you cross your legs into the butterfly position, you are effectively forcing proper form by not allowing your hip flexors to contract. It is also easy to modify in both directions to increase or decrease difficulty, which makes it perfect for group training sessions. I usually suggest this abs exercise to every client.

How to carry out:

• When you lie face up with your feet together, your knees should be bent out to the sides.

• Raise your arms over your head. This is the starting place.

• Using your core, roll your body up until you are sat upright.

• Reach out and touch your toes with your front arm.

• Start the following rep immediately after making a slow return to the starting position.

4. A LIFELESS BUG

A dead bug is the perfect way to stimulate the mind-muscle connection, which is necessary to stabilise and develop the various core muscles. The lovely thing about this exercise is that it builds core stability, which is crucial for day-to-day functioning, in addition to strengthening the transverse abdominis and spinal erectors.

Since the dead bug motion involves anti-extension, your goal should be to tighten your abdominal muscles in order to stop your lumbar spine from extending. It teaches superior form and technique for squats and deadlifts.

How to carry out:

• Assume a face-up position, extend your arms towards the sky, and arrange your legs in a tabletop stance, with your knees bent 90 degrees and stacked over your hips. This is the starting place.

• Slowly stretch your right leg straight while lowering your left arm to your side.

• Maintain a few inches of elevation between the two of you.

• Squeeze your butt while keeping your core stable and your lower back on the ground.

• Put your arm and leg back in the starting positions.

• Repeat on the other side, stretching your left and right legs this time.

5. CUTTING WOOD WITH HALF-KNEELING

Many people do not get the essential training in the transverse, or rotating, plane. It is very beneficial and tones your transverse abs, shoulders, and obliques.

How to carry out:

• While maintaining your foot level on the ground and your knee bent 90 degrees, take a few steps forward with one leg while kneeling.

• Hold a light to medium dumbbell with your leg bent towards the floor.

• Grab the weight firmly at both ends. This is where you should start.

• While bending your abs, lift the weight diagonally upward and towards the ceiling on the other side of your body.

• Keep your hips pointing forward; just your core muscles should rotate.

• Put the weight back where it was before.

• Finish all of your repetitions on one side, then switch to the other.

6. BOAT TO BOAT: LOW TO HIGH

This exercise strengthens the rectus abdominis, erector spinae, and hip flexors. What sustains my interest and involvement is the ongoing challenge.

How to carry out:

• Place your feet level on the floor and maintain a straight back.

• Carefully lift your legs off the ground until they are at a 45-degree angle with respect to your torso, keeping your alignment in mind.

• Keep your back flat, balance on your tailbone, and use your whole core.

• You may keep your knees bent (like in the picture) or straighten them out for a more difficult pose.

• Stretch your hands in front of you, it should be parallel to the floor.

• Place your hands under your hips if you feel like you need additional help.

- Hold for an additional three full breaths.

• After that, lower your upper body while extending your legs.

• A few inches above the floor should be the position of your shoulder blades and legs. If you find that too challenging, keep them raised off the ground slightly while you progressively lower them.

•After holding for a breath, raise your body and legs back to the High Boat.

7. DONNING A FOREARM ROCKER

You may improve your core strength and stability as well as your awareness of your body's various muscles by doing this exercise. Since this plank variation is undoubtedly tougher than a static plank, it's a great place to start building your core fitness. This exercise demonstrates the connection between your shoulders and core.

How to carry out:

• Start by putting your forearms on the floor, elbows directly behind your shoulders, palms facing forward so that your arms are parallel, and your legs extended behind you in the plank position.

• While tucking in your tailbone, flex your butt, quads, and core.

• Slightly bend your whole body forward such that your shoulders reach beyond your elbows and towards your hands.

• Take a few inches to recline.

• Take care to keep your quad, butt, and core engaged at all times.

8. BEND TO THE SIDE.

Throughout this exercise, your deep core muscles and obliques are worked. You'll also be strengthening your arms and back with this one. This is an exercise you can perform practically anywhere, including in your bedroom, and it will burn immediately.

How to carry out:

• Start in the side plank position, with your feet staggered as shown, your right hand precisely under your right shoulder, and your left foot squarely in front of your right.

As an alternative, you might position your left foot over your right.

• Tighten your core and butt. Let your left arm fall asleep by your side.

• After lowering your hips towards the floor, raise them back up.

• Finish all of your repetitions on one side, then switch to the other.

9. STAGGERED ROW WITH RESISTANCE BANDS

Since we utilise our core muscles more while standing, it's important to strengthen those muscles even though many core exercises are done on the floor. This practise may help you develop stability while strengthening your core.

How to carry out:

• Step with your left foot in front of your right to create a staggered posture. Extend your stance to make this position more comfortable.

• Loop the resistance band under your left foot, holding one end of it in each hand.

• Bend forward at the hips with your left leg slightly bent and your back straight.

• When you extend your arms all the way down to your left foot, the hand should feel loose. There's where you start.

• Hold your elbows, forearms, and hands perpendicular to your ribs while you do a row.

• Return your arms to your starting position to complete the rep.

• Finish all of your reps on one side, then switch to alternate your forward-facing foot positions.

10. HANDSOME .

You must use all of your core muscle groups in order to complete this thorough core exercise and keep your balance.

How to carry out:

• Extend your arms close to your ears while lying faceup on the floor.

• Squeeze your abs so that your low back presses the ground. This is the starting place.

• To lift your legs and upper back off the ground, extend your hands forward to meet your feet, pointing your toes while simultaneously squeezing your thighs and glutes. Your body will form a V shape as a result.

• Maintain a taut core as you gradually lower yourself to return to your starting position.

11. FROM HOLLOW HOLD TO JACKKNIFE

If required, you may modify this advanced action by maintaining your knees bent at a 90-degree angle. It is demanding, portable, efficient, and adaptable.

How to carry out:

• While laying face up, raise your arms straight over your head and place them close to your ears. Tighten your abs to use your low back to press the floor.

• Point your toes, tense your thighs and glutes, and raise your legs off the floor.

• Raise your shoulders off the ground and keep your head in a neutral position to prevent straining your neck.

• Your body should resemble a banana, with your hips and low back the only parts that are in contact with the earth. You should also have your midback and legs raised. The starting position is this empty grip.

• Maintain the hollow posture for a maximum of ten seconds.

• Upon inhaling, extend your arms and legs to make a V-shape with your body. After then, slowly return to your hollow position.

12. ROCK OF HOLLOW BODY.

This works the whole core as well as the rectus abdominis, transverse abdominis, and obliques. It teaches you how to put your whole body under stress, is easy to progress, and has a strong ab engagement that translates to other exercises like pull-ups and push-ups.

How to carry out:

• While laying faceup, raise your arms straight over your head and place them close to your ears.Tighten your abs to use your low back to press the floor.

• Point your toes, tense your thighs and glutes, and raise your legs off the floor.

• Raise your shoulders off the ground and keep your head in a neutral position to prevent straining your neck.

• Your body should resemble a banana, with your hips and low back the only parts that are in contact with the earth. You should also have your midback and legs raised. This is the starting place.

• Tension-building rocking back and forth until your hands and feet are almost in contact with the floor.

• Go back to the starting position and hold if this is too difficult.

13. C-SLOPE .

An isometric hold is the most difficult part of a sit-up. You are exercising your abs when you consistently put them under stress. It's a safe position for your back to stay in since your tailbone is tucked in and your spine is extended.

How to carry out:

• Sit on your tailbone with your feet flat on the ground. Hold onto one of each leg just above the knee.

• Rotate your spine, tuck your tailbone, and begin lowering your torso back as if you were lowering your back after a sit-up.

• At around halfway, stop and hold (as in the figure above).

• Continue to engage your quads and core fully.

• For an extra difficulty, let go of your legs and merely hold your arms in front of you.

14. DEADLIFT USING A RESISTANCE BAND ON ONE LEG

Taking positions that allow various body parts to interact and cooperate is crucial when trying to build a stronger core. This requires us to move in the following ways: we must bend, turn, and stand. In three dimensions, motion is required.

How to carry out:

- While standing with your feet shoulder-width apart, place the band under your left foot.
- When you stand with your arm down, holding the end of the band with your right hand will cause tension in the band. (You may either grasp the other end of the band in your left hand or let it dangle freely on the floor.)
- Put your whole weight on your left foot by making a movement with it.

• Lean forward until your chest is parallel to the floor, tip forward, bend at the hips, and let your right foot to rise up straight behind you. Sustain a robust core to facilitate equilibrium.

- As you hinge, let your right arm naturally fall towards the floor to lessen the pressure in the band.
- Replant your right foot in the ground to return to the starting position.
- Complete all the repetitions on one side before moving on to the other.
-

15. WHEELCHAIR

This is one of the activities that really helps you establish a psychological connection to your inner self. If you are not totally engaged, aware, and present throughout the whole exercise, you might easily let your lower back handle most of the work. And there are many other things that may be used as tools for this.

It specifically targets the stabilising muscles in your shoulders and abdomen, making it quite challenging.

How to carry out:

- Start on all fours, placing a glider or towel under each hand.
- Tighten your abs and tuck your tailbone to create a flat back, just as you would if you were doing a plank from your knees. This is the starting place.
- As you gradually bring your hands forward, maintain a straight posture.
- Glide as far as you can while maintaining a plank stance.
- Press into the ground and raise your arms to return to the starting position.

16. MOTION LIKE A BALL

This is a great aerobic workout that also works well for strengthening your core. While you swing back and forth, think on controlling it all from your abdomen.

How to carry out:

- With your knees bent and your feet forward, sit up.
- Wrap your arms over your legs and hold onto the outside of your ankles.
- Curl your head and chest forward so that they face your knees.
- Once your shoulders are in contact with the floor, roll back while firmly contracting your abdominal muscles.
- Wait until your head or neck touches the floor before turning over.
- Rock yourself back to your position.

17. LEG LIFTS

This exercise strengthens and lengthens the hip flexors, which are important for core stability and strength. It also works the lower abdominal area.

Along your fitness journey, your hip mobility will increase and benefit you in ways beyond just strengthening your abs. Incorporating them can improve your hip flexor flexibility since tight hip flexors are common, especially if you work a desk job all day.

How to carry out:

- Lay faceup with your hands at your sides or tucked under your hips for further support.
- Lift your legs gently, keeping them as straight and together as possible, until the soles of your shoes point upward.Then, softly spread your legs apart once again.
- Instead of letting your feet touch the ground, keep them hovering a few inches above it.

- As you do this movement, keep your lower back level on the ground. If you're having problems lowering your legs to that position, shorten the distance you lower them.

18. A BREAKDANCER

This exercise emphasises on possessing the strength to resist outside influences while trying to move your trunk. These improve your ability to change directions quickly and to accelerate and decelerate as well as your overall motor control.

How to carry out:

- Place your hands and knees under your shoulders and hips to begin on all fours.
- Lift your knees just a little bit off the ground.Stretch your right leg out from under you as you rotate your torso to the left, keeping your butt low.
- Extend your left arm in front of you.
- When you start to feel comfortable with the exercise and want a little more challenge with your balance, extend your arm out to tap your right foot.
- Return to your starting location after doing the same on the other side.

19. LEAN FORWARD ON A TABLE.

This exercise is really helpful if you have a split abdominal wall, back issues, or simply difficulty connecting with your core. That which I call a "core connector" It is recommended to be one of the first things to do when you get up in the morning.

How to carry out:

- Laying faceup with your legs up in a tabletop position, stack your knees over your hips.
- Tighten your abs to use your low back to press the floor.
- Put your hands on the front of your quads after doing a little crunch.

- Press your hands into your quadriceps as you push them away Your body should feel taut and in a battle, even if there shouldn't be any visible movements.

20. ROW YOUR BOAT!

With this exercise, you can definitely feel your oblique muscles working, and it gives the tactile sensation of strength.

How to carry out:

- Sit up straight with your legs bent and your feet flat on the floor.
- With your legs together, slowly lift them off the ground so that they form a 45-degree angle with your torso.
- Keep your back flat, use your whole core, and keep your weight on your tailbone.
- Your knees may be kept bent or straightened for a more challenging pose.
- Make sure your arms are parallel to the ground and straight out in front of you.
- If you think you need extra support, place your hands under your hips on the ground. It is known as High Boat.
- Clasp your hands in front of you and turn your waist to one side from this posture.
- Then, as if you were rowing with an oar in each hand, swing your arms to the same side.
- Quickly twist to the other side and repeat with your arms.
- Change sides all the time.

21. SIMPLE ROLL-UP

This method is requires you to start from a fully extended stance, which causes you to utilise much more of your core and less of your momentum to rise off the floor. Another challenge in this scenario is to keep your heels on the ground

How to carry out:

- With your feet flat on the floor and your arms lifted above your head, lie on your back.
- Float your arms up until your wrists are directly above your shoulders while you gradually elevate your spine off the floor, starting at your shoulders and working your way down to your lower back.
- Maintaining a firm core, sit up straight and then fold your body over your legs.
- To return to the earth, roll in the other direction, from your lower back to your shoulders.

22. A SINGLE JACKKNIFE

It works the rectus abdominis and, since you're reaching across your torso, it also works the obliques. It might also be altered. You may advance to a crunch with only one leg and then finish a sit-up. Before long, you'll be doing full V-ups with both arms and legs up at the same time, having mastered the single-arm, single-leg combo. Jacques

How to carry out:

- Lay faceup with your arms by your sides.
- Tighten your abs to use your low back to press the floor. This is the starting place.
- Raise your left leg and upper back off the ground, squeeze your glutes and thighs together, and move your right hand forward to meet your left foot.
- With your left leg and body, form a V.
- Maintain your core as you gradually refuse to return to your starting position.
- Proceed with the opposite limb and limb. Change sides all the time.

22. TAPE SHOULDER PLANK

This exercise aims to withstand rotation at the centre. To keep your hand off the ground and maintain alignment, your core must be engaged. Your hips should be totally stable, and your belly button should be towards the floor.

When compared to workouts that require you to lie down, like crunches or sit-ups, this particular exercise incorporates a lot more stability training. This implies that you are strengthening your back, shoulders, glutes, and hamstrings in addition to your abs. It might be easier or harder only by adjusting the width or length of your foot.

How to carry out:

- Beginning in a high plank position, place your hands shoulder-width apart, stack your shoulders over your wrists, extend your legs behind you, and maintain a taut core and glutes.
- While you tap your right hand on your left shoulder, keep your hips as stable as possible by using your core and glutes.
- Don't wag your hips.
- In the same way, touch your right shoulder with your left hand.
- PChange sides all the time.

24. KNEE DIVE

Through the tightening and strengthening of the transverse abdominis and obliques, this exercise strengthens and supports the whole core.

How to carry out:

- To start a forearm plank, place your forearms on the floor, your elbows should be directly beneath your shoulders, your hands should be pointed forward so that your arms are parallel, and your legs should be extended behind you.
- Tuck your tailbone in and contract your quadriceps, butt, and core.
- Turn your hips to the left and tap the floor. Repeat on the right side.
- Change sides all the time.

25. FOREARM PLANK COMBINED WITH LEG LIFT

By performing this exercise, whatever instability you can achieve will engage the deep abdominal muscles that surround your hips, spine, and reach your shoulders. Elevating your leg in a plank pose creates instability and works your glutes, which supports your lower back.

How to carry out:

- Starting on your hands and knees, lower yourself into a squat until your forearms are parallel to each other, your elbows exactly beneath your shoulders, and your palms and fingers facing forward.
- When you raise your knees off the floor and step your feet back, your legs should be straight and fully extended.
- Refrain from hunching your back and keep your quads, butt, and core firm. Consider length; picture yourself reaching from your heels to the top of your head at the same time.
- Maintain a neutral neck position by turning your head to face the floor.
- Tension your abdominals and raise one foot off the floor.
- After going back to the starting position, repeat on the other side. It is a single rep.
- Keep on switching.

26. DOG-BIRD

This exercise focuses on your core while you make use of one arm and the opposite leg at the same time. Walking in that manner is a terrific way to duplicate what we do every day, which makes it an even more effective exercise.

How to carry out:

- Assume a tabletop position on your hands and knees, placing your wrists under your shoulders and your knees under your hips.
- Stretch your left leg back and your right arm forward while keeping your back flat and your hips level with the floor.
- Think about placing your foot on the wall at your back. Just briefly uphold.
- Contract your abs as you return your arm and leg to their starting positions.
- Proceed with the opposite limb and limb. It is a single rep.
- Reps continue to be done while swapping sides.

27. PLANK ON THE SIDE WITH ARMS

Side planks work on muscles that are sometimes overlooked, such your glute medius, as well as spine stabilisers like the quadratus lumborum. These muscles help to keep your pelvis level while you're in a single-leg stance, which is basically where you are in a running stride most of the time. Since many running problems are linked to weakness, especially in the side hip stabiliser muscles, targeting these muscles with lateral planks is a smart way to cure this.

How to carry out:

- As you support your body on your right forearm, lay on your right side with your elbow stacked under your shoulder and your hand in front of your chest.
- After extending your legs and placing your left foot on top of your right, tighten your core and glutes to lift your hips off the ground.

- Holding your left hand vertically and pointing upward is the proper position.
- Sustain this alignment.
- Then alternate sides once more.

28. HEAVIER DEADLIFT

A deadlift works not just the lower body but also the transverse abdominis, rectus abdominis, erector spinae, and the internal and external obliques. A functional exercise that works muscles far deeper than the surface, the deadlift improves posture and overall strength while reducing the risk of lower back issues.

How to carry out:

- Relax your arms by your front quadriceps while standing with your feet hip-width apart, your knees slightly bent, and weights in each hand.
- From your hips, hinge forward, bending your knees slightly, push your butt all the way back, and keep your back flat.
- Gradually drop the weight along your shins.
- Your upper body ought to be almost parallel to the floor.
- Keeping your core firm, push through your heels to stand up straight and return to the starting position. Keep your weight close to your shins as you pull.
- Stop and squeeze your butt at the top.

29. OWN A BOAT.

This exercise is comparable to the plank since it is also an isometric that works the rectus and transversus abdominis as well as the internal and external obliques.

How to carry out:

- Sit up straight with your legs bent and your feet flat on the floor.
- With your legs together, slowly lift them off the ground so that they form a 45-degree angle with your torso.
- Keep your back flat, use your whole core, and keep your weight on your tailbone.
- Your knees may be kept bent (as in the picture) or straightened for a more challenging pose.
- Make sure your arms are parallel to the ground and straight out in front of you.
- If you think you need extra support, place your hands under your hips on the ground.
- Sustain this alignment.

30. FLYING UP A MOUNTAIN CLIMB

When done fast, this core exercise may help enhance cardiovascular health in addition to improving stability. Furthermore, since you have to utilise your core muscles constantly to move the glider back and forth, this version demands more core activity than mountain climbers without gliders.

How to carry out:

- Starting in a high plank position, place your hands shoulder-width apart (or wider if that's how you normally do push-ups), place your wrists over your shoulders, and place your toes on some gliders.
- Keeping your core stable, slide your right foot forward and pull your right knee up to your chest.
- As you advance your left foot and bring your right foot back, bring your left knee up to your chest.
- Alternatively, go at a fast pace.

- Keep your back flat at all times, and keep your core engaged.
- Go faster for a more intense aerobic workout. If you find it difficult to maintain your form, slow down.

31. HAVE A BAG WITH YOU

To avoid lateral flexion, or bending to one side, throughout this exercise, you must contract your core. It works wonders for strengthening the core. Tighten your core muscles to the maximum extent possible in order to resist gravity's pull to the side and keep your balance.

How to carry out:

- You want to position a dumbbell or kettlebell next to one of your feet.
- To pick up the weight, squat and use a neutral, palms-in hold.
- Maintain a firm core and an elevated chest as you stand up.
- As you go, resist the urge to wobble to one side in an attempt to balance the weight by keeping your body straight.
- Imagine yourself being pulled upward by a thread that is fastened to the top of your head.
- When finished, squat to return the weight to the ground. Repeat on the opposite side.

31. DRAWER-THROUGH BOARD

This is an excellent exercise programme to strengthen core stability and counter-rotation and anti-extension. This is one of the best and most intricate plank

How to carry out:

- Assume a high plank position by stretching your legs behind you wider than hip-width apart (this will help with stability), placing your hands shoulder-width apart, stacking your shoulders exactly above your wrists, and using your core and glutes.

- One palm should be slightly below a dumbbell. This is where it all started.
- With your hand facing away from the dumbbell, reach across your body, grab it, and pull it to the other side.
- Put your hand down on the ground in front of it once again.
- Keep your core stable to prevent swaying from side to side.
- Continue alternating after replicating on the opposite side.

34. BODIES WITH HOLES

Your deep core muscles and lower back will benefit greatly from this workout. Since it also helps with stability and posture, it's beneficial for those who need to strengthen their core to get rid of lower back stiffness. Beginners may do this exercise, and it can be modified to any degree of fitness by increasing or decreasing the difficulty.

How to carry out:

- With your arms over your head and close to your ears, lie on your back on a mat.
- Tighten your abdominal muscles to press your lower back on the floor.
- Point your toes, tense your thighs and glutes, and raise your legs off the floor.
- To raise your arms without straining your neck, elevate your shoulders off the floor while maintaining a neutral head posture.
- Just your lower back and hips should be in contact with the ground, forming the shape of a banana.
- You should also have your midback and legs raised.
- Sustain this alignment.

CHAPTER FOUR

REBUTTING THE MYTHS ABOUT CORE AND PROVIDING ANSWERS TO FREQUENTLY ASKED QUESTIONS ABOUT CORE EXERCISES

CORE AND PREGNANCY

Alot of people are confused on whether core exercises are good for pregnant women.

Maintaining a strong core during pregnancy is crucial for reducing back discomfort, and will also aid with labour, delivery, and recovery.

 Although this is true, there are several considerations when doing core exercises that must be taken carefully in order to prevent things like "diastasis recti" from becoming worse, which may cause problems for you postpartum and beyond.

REMEMBER THE FOLLOWING WHEN EXERCISING WHILE PREGNANT:

It's acceptable if you didn't work out before becoming pregnant! You may begin at any moment, but you should start out slowly and gauge your reaction to avoid overdoing it.

If it feels acceptable, you may maintain your regular exercise regimen throughout the first trimester.

It is advised to start reducing the intensity of your workouts in the second and third trimesters and to start changing things like supine core exercises, leaping, and high impact activities.

After the first trimester, it is not advised to do workouts while laying on your back for extended periods of time.

Avoid working out when it's too hot or humid since it could raise your body temperature and create dehydration or other negative effects.

Avoid overdoing certain abdominal workouts since doing so might raise pressure in the core, particularly in the obliques.

Exercises involving quick movements, twists, or turns should be avoided.

BEST ABSORBING CORE EXERCISES TO DO WHILE PREGNANT

Caution: Before beginning, get medical advice.

It is really helpful to keep exercising and being active during your pregnancy. You may do the following workouts while pregnant:

KNEELIFT WHILE SEATED

Sit in a chair, perch on the edge of your sofa, or use an exercise ball.

How to:

- Sit close to the chair's edge.

- Just under your knees, keep your feet firmly planted on the ground.
- Maintain downward-facing palms under your hips.
- Bend your left leg so that it tilts your pelvis and activates your pelvic floor, then slowly compress your abdomen.
- Then, as you breath, carefully raise your left knee to your chest.
- Take a breath in and bring your left foot back to the floor to resume your starring posture.
- Continue by using your right leg.
- Do 2-3 sets of 8–12 repetitions. You may also add little weights (2 to 5 pounds) to each ankle during the first trimester.

THE SIDE-LYING CRUNCH

How to:

- Lay down on the rug or floor.
- Bend your knees at a 30 degree angle to your hips while slowly rolling to the left.
- Your knees should be roughly 6 inches off the ground as you roll your torso to the right.
- Make sure the left shoulder blade and the rear of the shoulder are supported by your body weight.
- Put your hands behind your head, fingers touching, but avoid pulling your neck.
- As if you were reaching for your right knee, diagonally curl your body upward. As high as you can, raise.
- Your left shoulder will slightly elevate off the floor as you do the aforementioned motions.
- Curl your arms a little higher as you bring them up to your knees.
- After then, put your hands behind your head and return to your starting posture.
- Do the same on the other side.
- Execute two sets of 10–12 repetitions on each side.

CORE RESPIRATION

This core workout is incredibly simple yet powerful.

- How to:
- Standing or sitting comfortably while maintaining a straight back.
- Place one hand on your chest and the other on your waist or tummy.
- Inhale deeply for roughly 5 to 10 counts, feeling your ribcage widen.
- As you exhale, count to five to ten before bringing your ribs back together.
- By tensing the front of your pelvis and the back of your tailbone, you may relax your muscles.
- Ten deep breaths should be taken repeatedly.

THE SEATED BALL'S STABILITY

On an exercise ball instead of the ground, this activity is comparable to bird dog.

How to:

- Sit upright and tall on a stability ball.
- To keep your balance, place hands on both of your sides.
- Take a deep breath in as you lift your right foot off the floor and extend your left arm upward.
- After holding for two to three seconds, return to the beginning position.
- Redo again using the left foot and right arm.
- 2–3 rounds of 10 on each side are ideal.

SIDE LUNGE/MODIFIED SIDE LUNGE

There are various variations of the side plank. These are some possibilities you have when pregnant.

How to:

- Place your elbow beneath your shoulder while starting on your side.
- When stacking the knees, keep one straight, one bent, or straight out if it feels comfortable. Avoid coning.
- Focus on your core breathing while maintaining a neutral spine and a flat back.
- Keep your head and neck straight and squeeze your hips and lift your body to form a straight line from head to hips.
- Remain in the posture for 20 to 30 seconds while breathing.
- On the other side, repeat.

THE STANDING CRUNCH

This is a safe crunch that is similar to one you might make when laying down.

How to:

- Standing upright, place your hands behind your head, knees slightly bent, and feet hip width apart
- Inhale Tuck your pelvis in and draw your belly button in.
- Exhale, then crunch forward while contracting your abdominal muscles in the same manner as you would if you were laying on your back.
- Intend to do 15–20 repetitions.

THE UPRIGHT BICYCLE

This is a great workout for strengthening your core and improving balance.

How to:

- Standing with your feet hip-width apart and your hands behind your head, breathe in

- Next, exhale. While you crunch, bring your left elbow to rest on top of your right knee.
- Replicate it with your left foot and right elbow while returning to your starting standing posture.
- Attempt 10–20 reps.

KEGELS

How to:

- Place your feet comfortably on the exercise ball and take a deep breath. Allow your tummy to expand as you take in air as you inhale. Once you've taken in enough breath, softly exhale to let the remaining air out.
- Try to match your inhale length (5–10) to your exhalation length (5–10).
- Try to tense your vaginal muscles the next time you breath. It should mirror the muscles contracting when you really need to urinate but are compelled to keep it in.
- Relax your shoulders, face, and neck. Only the pelvic floor muscles should feel tight and constricted at this time. Hold the position for five to eight counts, then release gradually.
- To gradually raise the number, try to perform this 20 times every day.

SQUAT

Some people may not be aware that if performed properly, this exercise can help you strengthen your abdominal muscles and be ready for the pushing phase of delivery.

How to:

- Stand up with your feet apart from your hips.
- Straighten your arms and raise them over your chest.
- As you crouch down, breathe in and put weight on your heels to prevent your knees from collapsing.
- Exhale as you pause at the bottom and raise to a standing posture.

- Do two or more sets of 15 repetitions.

COW AND CAT POSE

Your back and spine will be more flexible as a result of this, which also serves to develop your core muscles.

How to:

- Begin in tabletop position on the floor with your hands immediately behind your shoulders and your knees directly beneath your hips.
- Inhale, raise your head, arch your back, and let your stomach hang.
- Inhale, tuck your chin and tailbone in, and bring your belly towards your spine as you exhale.
- Continue practising the inhaling and exhaling exercise until you can, as closely as possible, match the rhythm of your breathing to the rhythm of your movements.
- The steps should be repeated for around two minutes, followed by a rest.

SIDE-LYING LEG RAISES

It aids in building up your glute, hip, and core muscles.

How to:

- Legs placed one on top of the other, lie on your left side. So that it can support your upper body, keep your left elbow on the floor.
- Now carefully elevate your right leg or both of your legs (advanced and more only first trimester). As high as you can, raise it. Make certain that your hips are parallel to your torso.
- Lower your right leg till it is two inches or less over your left leg.

- 20 repetitions should be completed with each leg, and you should continue until your legs begin to feel exhausted.

DOG BIRD CRUNCHES

This stability workout will make your abs stronger.

How to:

- Start off in a tabletop posture with your back straight, knees under your hips, and wrists exactly behind your shoulders.
- Hold your core tight as you gently inhale, raise your left leg and stretch it behind you in a straight line, and lift your right arm straight up in front of you.
- Exhale bring the left knee to the centre of the right elbow.
- Breathe in, exhale, then repeat for 10–12 times.
- Next, repeat the process with the hand and leg on the other side of you.

PELVIC TILT WHEN STANDING

It is a beneficial workout to strengthen your back and abdominal muscles as well as to help you stand more straight.

How to:

- Place your back and hips on the wall while you stand straight next to it.
- Your lower back will have a slight gap between it and the wall.
- Then tilt your pelvis while tightening your abs. The hips Your lower back should flatten against the wall as you do this.
- Try to accomplish this stance 10 times while holding it for five seconds, then releasing it.

A HIP HIKER

The hip and glute muscles are strengthened as a result.

Ways to:

Easily recline on your side.

Keep your upper leg straight while bending your lower leg. Make use of a cushion to support your head if you're uncomfortable.

Now lift your upper leg off the floor by two to four inches.

Maintain a straight leg. Pulling your hip requires using the muscles on the side of your abdomen.

For around five seconds, maintain the posture.

Ten times through the process.

HEEL SLOSHING

How to:

Begin in a glute bridge posture on the floor.

Extend one leg at a time, lifting your heel just a tiny bit off the ground.

Return to your starting position gradually. (Can be carried out with a glider or a towel under the heel)

Continue with the opposite

CORE AND BELLY FAT

This will provide an insight on what belly fat is and core workouts for belly fat

How Abdominal Fat Affects Health And What It Is

Your body has two different forms of fat: visceral fat and subcutaneous fat. You may reach out and grasp the subcutaneous fat that is located just under your skin. Visceral fat, which is located deeper in your stomach, is considered abdominal fat.

Health is directly impacted by visceral fat, which is the fat that surrounds your abdominal organs. For instance, it may impair how the body reacts to insulin, resulting in elevated levels of both blood sugar and insulin. Additionally, it may result in heart disease and excessive cholesterol. Therefore, your waistline is more significant than your weight on the scale.

This is due to your body's organs being overrun by free fatty acids from visceral fat, which the cells are unable to process. There may be a number of health issues as a consequence.

You may be more susceptible to heart attacks, heart disease, stroke, insulin resistance, diabetes, and several malignancies if visceral fat accumulates around the waist. Visceral fat may have a variety of effects since it surrounds the organs and is located deep inside the stomach's cavity.

For instance, the liver converts fat into all the many forms of cholesterol found in the body. Normal quantities of fat and cholesterol are essential to the body because they help create bile, which is required to absorb fat and fat-soluble vitamins from meals, as well as hormones and human cells. LDL, or bad cholesterol, builds up in arteries when blood levels are too high, which causes the arteries to stiffen and constrict. Atherosclerosis is the term for this.

Additionally, abdominal obesity may cause insulin resistance, which can turn into type 2 diabetes. The amount of visceral fat present is a more important determinant than being overweight. While technically overweight individuals do not, some persons with extra fat and a normal BMI do.

Additionally, it has been shown that retinol-binding protein 4 levels above normal increase insulin resistance. This protein is secreted by visceral fat, which is how having more of this specific fat raises your risk.

How to Lose Belly Fat

- Through Nutrition
- Through Exercise

HOW TO LOSE BELLY FAT THROUGH CORE EXERCISES

If you want to effectively decrease and avoid visceral fat, think about include regular exercise in your routine in addition to your diet. But bear in mind that you usually can't focus on only your stomach. Instead, the workouts you do will lower your overall body fat.

In exercise, lowering fat in a specific location, such as the waist, is known as spot reduction. Exercise may often decrease abdominal adiposity, or extra belly fat, but it's impossible to exclusively lose fat in one part of the body at a time. You need a comprehensive workout schedule.

For instance, following a 12-week fitness programme, participants in one research saw a reduction in abdomen fat. They used a bicycle for 45 minutes each time they worked out.

CORE AND BLOATING

Can doing core workouts make you bloated

Nothing improves our mood like a good exercise. There is gushing perspiration. Even though we are exhausted, we feel energised because endorphins are being released. Both physically and symbolically, we are fired up.

But have you ever experienced post-workout bloating? Have you ever felt sluggish and bloated rather than trim and elegant? If so, you are not alone yourself. The post-workout bloat is a common phenomena that affects lots of individuals.

You could be curious as to why it occurs and if it's typical. Here is all the information you want about post-workout bloating.

Is feeling bloated after working out normal?

The simple answer is yes, feeling bloated after working out is normal.

Why? Well, if you've been exhaling quickly or drinking too much water, which might lead you to swallow air, you could feel bloated after a workout. Exercise may result in bloating on its own, and if you overhydrate or don't drink enough, you could feel stomach distension.

Several factors might contribute to post-workout bloating, post-workout bloating is typical, but it t usually isn't a reason for alarm.

What Results In Bloating After Exercise?

You could feel bloated during or after a workout for a variety of reasons, including:

DEHYDRATION

Although it may sound weird, dehydration, or a lack of fluids, is the primary cause of bloating. Why? Your stomach holds water to make up for a lack of fluid in your body, which causes outward swelling. Drinking extra water is the most effective strategy to remove the edoema.

OVERHYDRATION

Hyponatremia, a disease where your body dilutes its sodium concentration and causes your cells to retain water, may be brought on by consuming too much water too rapidly.

NUTRITION

Eating too soon before going to the gym might make you bloated even though you want to fuel your body for your exercise, especially if you want to undertake a lengthy bike, run, or other high intensity activity. This is particularly true if your meal has a lot of fat, fibre, or protein.

If you eat right before exercising, your body will struggle to multitask digesting food and sending blood to your working muscles. The germs in your digestive system may react to delayed digestion by producing some gas, which may cause you to feel bloated.

HEAT

You can experience belly bloating or swelling when it's really hot outdoors or you're exercising in a warm, stuffy atmosphere. That's because heat makes your blood vessels enlarge, which might result in fluid building up between tissues.

Try exercising in an air-conditioned space while wearing breathable, lightweight training attire to help prevent heat-related bloating.

EXERTION

Exercise is challenging. After all, there's a purpose for the term "working out." But as your body starts to heal itself, you could feel bloated or inflamed. This is a typical procedure that is critical to healing.

"If you eat right before exercising, your body will struggle to multitask digesting food and sending blood to your working muscles," says board-certified physician. The germs in your digestive system may react to delayed digestion by producing some gas, which may cause you to feel bloated.

A LOT OF BREATHING

When you exercise, it's natural for your respiratory rate to rise. Your body produces more carbon dioxide and needs more oxygen while you exercise. However, sucking in a lot of air during an exercise might happen if you breathe too forcefully.

The air can make its way down into your digestive system instead of going straight to your lungs. You'll feel bloated and puffy when this happens."

HOW SHOULD I HANDLE POST-WORKOUT BLOATING?

Although post-workout bloating is unpleasant, the symptom is temporary. Discord and inflammation brought on by exercise often disappear on their own. But if you want to calm your stomach and get rid of your symptoms, think about trying these remedies:

EAT SENSIBLY.

While certain meals are healthier than others, it's important to know what to eat before and after exercise. Stick to basic carbohydrates and easier-to-digest proteins, Greek yoghurt, eggs, and pasta are all excellent options.

DRINK ENOUGH WATER.

Your body loses salt and electrolytes while you exercise because you sweat. However, drinking water before to and after an exercise will aid in your body's recovery and return of its normal fluid balance. Not sure how much liquid you should consume? weigh oneself before and after exercising. For every pound lost, you should generally consume three glasses of water.

Steer clear of soda, alcohol, and meals high in sugar. Although it's crucial to know what to eat after an exercise, your recovery and digestive health depend on you also knowing what to avoid.

Avoid soda and alcohol since they can contribute to or exacerbate bloating. It's preferable to stick to the fundamentals and avoid fried meals altogether if possible. Avoid foods that are greasy, sweet, or fibrous.

HOW CAN I AVOID BLOATING AFTER EXERCISE?

Although post-workout bloating may be treated, avoiding it altogether is the best approach to handle it. Making ensure your body is prepared for exercise is a key component of prevention.

Eat a meal two to three hours before doing exercise to nourish your body and allow it time to digest the food.

Drinking water 30 to 60 minutes before doing out can help you prevent feeling bloated. If you're going to consume water while working out, sip it more slowly. Bloating may result from consuming too much water in a short amount of time.

Controlling your breathing. "As you workout, maintain slow, even breathing. Avoid gasping or taking deep breaths.

You may also take supplements. "Taking a good postbiotic supplement can optimise digestion, helping to minimise post-workout bloating," O.

The conclusion

Bloating after exercise is pretty typical. Additionally, it may be quite unpleasant. The illness may cause a variety of uncomfortable symptoms, including gas and bloating as well as an overall sense of fullness.

Thankfully, post-workout bloating is temporary. Its symptoms may be reduced with a few preemptive steps and post-workout treatments, and it often goes away on its own.

CORE AND BACK PAIN

*Can core training lead to back discomfort

Why doing core exercises could cause lower back pain

BAD MANNERS

Poor form during ab exercises is the main contributor to lower back discomfort. For instance, back pain might result from using your back muscles instead of your abdominal ones. Another example is the excessive back curvature that might strain the lower spine while lifting.

These are excellent illustrations of the reasons why doing core workouts might cause lower back discomfort in certain individuals.

Too Soon And Too Much

Even with proper technique, doing several ab exercises too soon might cause lower back discomfort.

If you don't gradually concentrate on building the ab muscles over time, exercising too hard or for too long might cause weariness and back discomfort.

Heating Up

Before doing exercise, warming up or stretching helps get your body ready by triggering your muscles and boosting blood flow.

Unengaged muscles may not be ready for strenuous motions, which might result in lower back pain and injury.

Another factor contributing to lower back discomfort during ab workouts is being out of shape. Your muscles experience stress and strain from regular exercise, which over time helps you gain strength and confidence. It is ensured that you don't overlook any muscles by subjecting the body to a variety of activities.

You are only as powerful as your weakest link in the chain that is your body. The lower back may have to work too hard or may not be able to support the weight if certain parts are not strong enough. Make sure you are consistently engaging in a variety of workouts.

HOW TO AVOID LOWER BACK INJURIES WHILE DOING ABDOMINAL EXERCISES

Warm-ups

When pushed for time, it may be tempting to omit the pre-workout warm-up. To prepare your muscles for the effort ahead, ease into the exercise with moderate stretches or progressive motions. It facilitates muscular activation and boosts blood flow.

Spend 10 to 15 minutes doing easy exercises like lunges, shoulder rolls, and moderate trunk rotations. If you feel pain, stop.

Stop working out right away if your back begins to ache, and write down what caused it. Exercise-related discomfort is a strong indication that you should reconsider your training schedule.

Exercises that could be causing your discomfort should be avoided or changed. As an alternative, you can think about seeing a health expert like a physical therapist or strength coach.

Developing your lower back and core muscles

You may protect your lower back during abdominal exercises by strengthening or exercising your lower back muscles more often. This is especially true if you have a sedentary work schedule and poor posture.

Lower back discomfort may result from even easy workouts like brisk walking if the muscles are weak or not functioning properly.

You may want to start with exercises like planks, bridges, dead bugs, and pelvic tilts. You may progressively increase your core strength with these exercises to guard against lower back problems.

Starting with simple motions before moving on to more difficult ones is another efficient strategy for preventing lower back discomfort during ab workouts.

While it may be tempting to experiment with more sophisticated methods, ailments like lower back discomfort are more likely to occur if you don't establish your basics.

HOW IMPROVING CORE STABILITY MAY REDUCE LOWER BACK PAIN

The muscles of the front abdominal region, such as the rectus abdominis, deep abdominal region, such as the transverse abdominis, side of the body, such as the obliques, quadratus lumborum, and back, such as the erector spinae, multifidus, etc., make up the core.

The diaphragm, gluteal muscles, and hip flexors are among the surrounding muscles that support the core.

The spine needs stability from the core in order to be protected against difficult or heavy motions.

What Happens If We Do Ab Exercises When Our Core Muscles Are Weak?

The passive structures in our body need support and protection, which is one of the core's main functions. The body's passive components, such as the joints, ligaments, and spinal discs, aren't the ones that start motions.

Lower back discomfort during ab exercises might be caused by weak core muscles. The vertebrae, ligaments, discs, and other components of the spine may not be as well protected from the stress and strain of ab exercises if your core muscles are not sufficiently developed.

EXERCISES TO BUILD CORE STRENGTH

There are various strategies to develop core strength, including:

Isometric workouts, such side planks and farmer's walks, maintain the core tight and firm

Dynamic workouts, such crunches and Russian twists, emphasise strengthening activities while the core moves.

Exercises For The Core To Avoid If You Have Lower Back Discomfort

Not all of these activities, but several of the more typical ones, may make lower back discomfort worse.

Lumbar flexion, which is necessary for sit-ups, puts strain on your spine. You may be able to separate your abdominal muscles with partial crunches without running the same danger.

Running, contact sports, trampolining, and snowboarding are examples of high-impact aerobics.

Extremely twisting activities, such as in golf, tennis, or yoga

Superman extensions for the back

Toe touches when standing

If your lower back hurts as you work on your abs, talk to a physical therapist or strength coach about switching up your training plan.

They could also assist in ensuring that you carry out the activity properly. The chance of lower back pain, discomfort, and other types of damage may be decreased by using the right technique.

These workouts strengthen your abdominal muscles more than crunches alone while safeguarding your back and neck.

DEAD BUGS:

Assume a prone position, raising your arms above, bending your knees to a 90-degree angle, and bending your hips. Breathe out deeply and extend the other person's arm and leg while keeping your rib cage low.

LEG LOWERING:

Assume a prone position once again and elevate your legs such that your feet point upward. Then, with one leg straight up as if you were standing on a hot cup of coffee, slowly lower the other leg as cl0ose to the ground as you can before raising it back to the starting position.

FRONT PLANK:

Avoid sagging or propping up your hips by beginning on your toes and elbows. Before the difficulty level is increased, the goal time should be about sixty seconds.

SIDE BOARD BAND ROW:

To increase the difficulty, do a row with your upper arm while clutching a band or cable.bending half way Pallof Press: Bend your inner knee while standing on one knee. Start at your closest heart-level and work your way out to a comfortable distance. Once that is done, straighten your arms while keeping your core still and avoiding spinning.

AB WHEEL ROLLOUTS:

Start on your knees, softly extend your arms, and maintain a flat lower back.

HOLLOW HOLDS:

Sit up" from a prone posture and raise your arms and legs. Lower your hands and feet only as much as necessary to keep your spine in its hollowed-out position.

CORE AND HERNIA

Can core training lead to hernias?

Hernias occur when an internal body component pushes through a weak spot in the muscle or tissue of the body. A hernia often develops between the chest and hips. At first, there are either little or no symptoms. However, you could detect a lump or bulge in your groyne or abdomen.

There are three different forms of hernias.

Inguinal hernia

When the bladder or bowel presses through vulnerable areas of the lower abdominal wall, an inguinal hernia results.

Hiatal Hernia:

Extra stomach tissue that pushes through the diaphragm may cause a hernia to form in the chest area. Smokers are more likely to develop this illness. Additionally linked to gastroesophageal reflux disease and acid reflux is a hiatal hernia.

Umbilical hernia:

This condition develops when a portion of the intestines pokes through the muscles of the abdomen around the belly button. The illness most often affects children and expectant mothers, although it may also afflict male adults.

Hernia and exercise. Are you sure?

Some individuals with hernias may be able to safely exercise. Exercise with a hernia could be safe, but you should proceed with care. Concentrate on tasks that won't put pressure on your hernia to avoid further damage. When dealing with abdominal hernias, it is not advised to conduct workouts or lift routines that strain or pull the abdominal region. However, there are a few workouts to stay away from. Knowing which workouts to avoid is the first step in exercising safely.

It's also a good idea to exercise with a certified physiotherapist or personal trainer. You may get safe workout advice from the trainer or physiotherapist. When you have been diagnosed with a hernia or are recuperating from a hernia procedure, talk to your doctor before exercising.

Exercise benefits for hernia:

There is some evidence to suggest that yoga or exercise might hasten or assist the recovery after hernia surgery. Physical therapists and doctors advise exercise and yoga for a healthy lifestyle. It's critical to comprehend your doctor's recommendations for the best workouts and the best time to start them.

1. **Core Strengthening:**

Weak core muscles are a common cause of hernias. By using your abdominal muscles and obliques during certain workouts and yoga positions, you may strengthen your abdominal wall.

2. **Activate smaller muscle fibres:**

Yoga poses, gentler workouts, and stretches may all target fascia, the fibrous web that surrounds your muscles. As you gain movement, your myofascial connective tissue helps maintain your organs in their proper positions.

3. Increase body awareness:

By linking your breath to your activity, you may better understand how you are feeling and where a discomfort could be located. Yoga is a great approach to bring balance back to the body for persons who are imbalanced or "stuck in their heads" who are feeling stress or worry.

4. A quicker recovery from surgery:

Research has shown that post-operative yoga lowers pain, side effects, and the risk of hernia recurrence.

Core Exercises for inguinal hernia recovery:

1. Pillow Squeeze:

To do the Pillow Squeeze, contract your thigh muscles. Start by bending your knees and resting flat on the ground. Holding a cushion between your legs, take a deep breath. Gently grasp the cushion with both legs as you exhale. Remember to do this workout 20 times per day.

2. Shoulder Bridge:

Sit with a cushion in between your knees and exhale while maintaining the same posture for your knees. To give support, raise your waist and place your arms on the ground. From your shoulders to your knees, try to maintain as much straightness as you can. Increase your breathing. Put a cushion between your knees and sit back down in your original posture. 20 times each day.

3. To stretch your hamstrings, bend your knees and lay flat on the ground. Your chin and head need to be at eye level. Then, lift one leg while maintaining the bend in the other. Try drawing the raised leg towards you while putting a towel over your foot. Your hamstring muscles should feel somewhat stretched when you attempt to stretch them. For

at least 30 seconds, maintain that posture. Then return to your starting point. Ten times a day, alternate between each leg.

4. Opening the knee:

As you lay flat on the floor, bend your knees and take a deep breath. Open one knee sideways and exhale. Bring it as near the ground as you can. Bring your knee back now. Apply the same technique to the opposite knee. Five times each day, repeat this. During the workout, keep your body in a straight posture.

5. Roll your hips:

While maintaining a wide stance, bend your knees the same way. Put your arms in front of you and, take a deep breath. As you shift to your right side and softly inhale, roll over your hips. Knees should be sideways bent. The opposing side should follow suit. Ten times a day, then 20 times a day, repeat this exercise.

Good core exercises for a hiatal hernia include:

1. Chair Pose:

The lower body and core are strengthened in this position. Put your feet together closely. Put your knees together and place your hands above your head. By bending the knees as far as you can, you should maintain your thighs parallel to the ground. Hold the stretch for as long as you can and then come back to the beginning position.

2. Bridge Position:

With this exercise, you may strengthen the muscles in your stomach. Knees bowed, lay on your back with both feet flat on the floor. Lift the lower back off the floor while keeping the shoulders down. As long as you can, hold this posture before shifting back to your starting position.

3. Diaphragmatic breathing:

It helps persons with hiatal hernias by strengthening the diaphragm. Either sit upright or lay down. Place on hand on your stomach while the other on your chest. Inhale deeply through your nostrils while paying attention to the rising of your stomach. Put your attention on lowering your stomach as you exhale through pursed lips. Do this many times.

Suitable core exercises for umbilical hernia

1. Cycling in the air:

By cycling your legs in the air, you may strengthen your lower abdominal muscles. Lie down on a slanted board. With slant boards, you may relieve extra strain off your feet and head while working out. By elevating your legs towards your chest, you may do cycling leg movements on your slant board. Holding your sides while cycling your legs can help you remain steady. Three times each week, spend 10 to 15 minutes doing these exercises.

2. Stretching:

To lower the danger of hernias, it's essential to have a flexible abdomen. Lay down on the ground with your knees bent straight. Legs bent on either side, strive to contact the surface while keeping your back firmly planted on the ground. After holding the position for 5 to 10 seconds, switch back to your beginning position. On the other side, repeat the process. This stretch should be done each day. By stretching them, your abdominal muscles become more flexible and are less prone to become weak under stress.

3. Adjust Your Breathing:

Correct breathing should always be used while exercising. Instead of breathing from your chest, take deep abdominal breaths. It raises the diaphragm, which aids in releasing abdominal pressure. Your back need to be flat on the floor. You should lay one hand on your tummy and the other on your chest. Breathe in via your nose, allowing air to enter your abdomen. As you breathe in, elevate your lower hand instead of the hand on your chest.

Exercise regimen after hernia surgery

Only after talking with the surgeon should you proceed.

Deep Breathing:

It's common to have some discomfort following surgery. Deep breathing may be quite unpleasant, especially after abdominal surgery, which causes patients to breathe very shallowly. Infections at the bottom of the lungs may sometimes result from an inability to expand the lungs correctly. Therefore, during the day, you should take a few mindful, deep breaths. To get rid of phlegm or sputum, you should also cough carefully. You may assist your cough by holding a cushion or cloth next to the surgical site. This will help you cough and empty your lungs appropriately.

Walking:

To hasten your recovery after hernia surgery, walking is a highly advised form of exercise. You promote healthy circulation and continued function of your intestines by doing this. Patients should walk a bit after surgery and then gradually increase their distance as they recuperate. Walking promotes healing more quickly and guards against blood clots and infection.

Leg exercises:

By keeping the blood flowing, leg workouts provide you the power to keep your legs flexible and avoid blood clots. Start by doing each exercise many times, then as your strength improves, increase the number of repetitions.

Ankle flex:

Alternate between stretching and flexing your ankles for ten repetitions.

Knee pushes:

While laying on your back, press your thigh up against the edge of the bed while holding for a few seconds and relaxing your muscles.

eg Straighten: While seated on the side of the bed, straighten your legs by bending your knees with your feet flat on the floor. One leg at a time, extend it straight for a moment, then bring it back to a 90-degree angle.

Abdominal workouts can strengthen your core muscles and lower your risk of hernias:

Lay on your back, bend your knees, and place your hands on your hips to do a button pull. Pull your belly button in while you take a deep breath in and out gently. Do this many times.

Core twists:

To ensure that your spine is stable, lie on your back with your legs bent and grip your hands on each side of your body. Kneel down on one side as far as you can while keeping your feet on the bed, then stand up straight. On the other side, repeat.

Pelvic tilts:

With your knees bent and your feet flat on the ground, place your hands beneath your lower back. Your bottom should be tilted forward, and your spine should be flattened on your hands. Return to the starting location after a brief interval.

Avoid these exercises after hernia surgery:

Following hernia surgery or if you have a hernia, you should refrain from engaging in certain workouts and activities:

1. You should refrain from engaging in painful exercise, such as weightlifting.

2. Refrain from excessive abdominal stretching. The abdominal muscles are overworked when they are exercised in methods that extend them, such as the yoga posture known as upward dog.

3. Steer clear of Pilates, planks, crunches, and other core-strengthening activities.

4. Steer clear of contact-heavy, high-impact exercises.

Key Learnings:

To ensure your safety when exercising while you have a hernia, keep the following advice in mind. Avoiding the hard workouts mentioned above is one of the most critical stages. Make sure to include aerobic workouts, glute bridges, and posture strengthening exercises into your training regimen

Make careful not to go too far. Till your hernia is fixed, you should be patient with yourself.

Exercise may help you manage your hernia more effectively and get you ready for surgery if that becomes required. It is unquestionably a crucial component of your preventative strategy after surgery.

When you start exercising, your hernias might potentially become worse. Therefore, patients must have hernia therapy before engaging in vigorous activity. Since every individual is unique, it is essential to discuss the best time to start exercising and the appropriate kind of exercise with your doctor.